Lift, Twist, Stand

Mastering the Turkish Get-Up

Helen Talbott

Disclaimer

The information provided in "Lift, Twist, Stand: Mastering the Turkish Get-Up" is intended for general informational purposes only. The author and publisher are not responsible for any injury, damage, or negative consequences resulting from the use of the exercises, techniques, or information presented in this book. Readers are advised to consult with a qualified healthcare professional or fitness expert before beginning any new exercise program, especially if they have pre-existing health conditions or concerns. The author and publisher are not responsible for any injury, damage, or negative consequences resulting from the use of the exercises, techniques, or information presented in this book. Readers are advised to consult with a qualified healthcare professional or fitness expert before beginning any new exercise program, especially if they have pre-existing health conditions or concerns. The author

Table of contents

About the Author

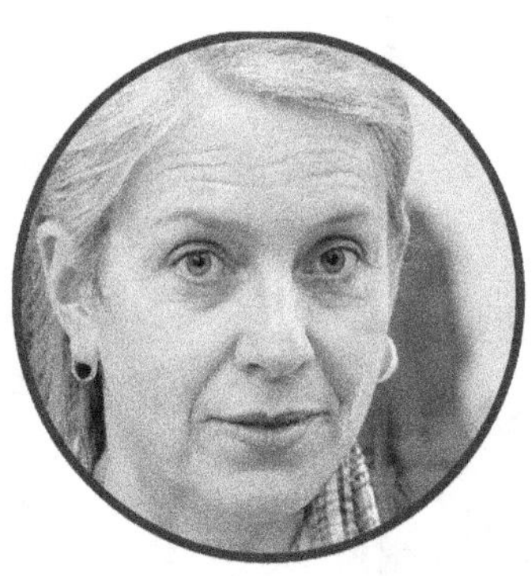 Helen Talbott, the creative mind behind this ab workout exercise book, brings a unique blend of passion for fitness and strategic thinking to the world of wellness. She has dedicated her expertise to helping individuals battle the bulge and achieve their fitness goals.

Helen Talbott is not just an author; she is a certified fitness instructor with a profound understanding of abdominal muscles and the science behind combating belly fat. Her commitment to a holistic approach to health and well-being is evident in the carefully crafted workouts and strategies presented in this book.

With a background in exercise science and years of hands-on experience in the fitness industry, Helen Talbott has become a trusted resource for those seeking effective and sustainable ways to enhance their core strength.
Through her writing, Helen Talbott aims to demystify the complexities of ab workouts, providing readers with actionable advice, personalized plans, and the motivation needed to combat belly fat successfully. Whether you're a fitness enthusiast or someone embarking on a wellness journey for the first time, Helen Talbott insights will guide you toward a stronger, healthier, and more confident you.

Introduction

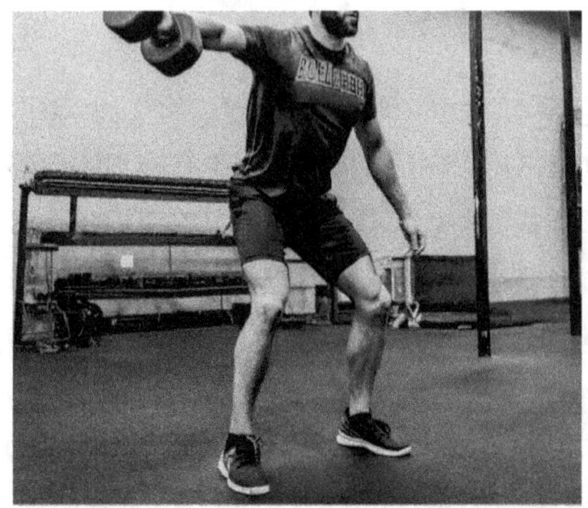

Welcome to "Lift, Twist, Stand: Mastering the Turkish Get-Up." This book is your comprehensive guide to unlocking the full potential of a timeless exercise that transcends fitness trends – the Turkish Get-Up.

The Turkish Get-Up, originating from the ancient tradition of Turkish wrestlers, has evolved into a cornerstone of modern functional fitness. Its elegance lies in its complexity, seamlessly integrating strength, mobility, and stability. Whether you are a seasoned athlete or a newcomer to the world of exercise, this book is designed to demystify the Turkish Get-Up, providing you with a structured pathway to mastery.

In the following chapters, we'll delve into the Lift, Twist, Stand principles that form the foundation of the Turkish Get-Up. From the nuanced body mechanics and alignment to the intricacies of initiating the movement, this guide breaks down each phase to enhance your understanding and execution. You'll find detailed explanations of the key muscles involved, common mistakes to avoid, and progressions tailored to your skill level.

As you embark on this journey, envision the Turkish Get-Up not merely as an exercise but as a holistic movement that fosters strength, flexibility, and mindfulness. Each page is crafted to empower you, offering insights, tips, and variations that cater to individual differences and goals.

Whether you aspire to build strength, improve endurance, or enhance your overall functional fitness, the Turkish Get-Up is a versatile tool that can be tailored to suit your aspirations. Get ready to embark on a transformative exploration of movement, where Lift, Twist, Stand become more than words – they become a roadmap to mastering the Turkish Get-Up and, by extension, your own physical potential.

Overview of the Turkish Get-Up

The Turkish Get-Up is a multi-phased, full-body exercise that transcends traditional fitness routines. This movement, rooted in strength training and functional fitness, requires a seamless combination of lifting, twisting, and standing. The overview delves into the fundamental principles behind the Turkish Get-Up, highlighting its significance in promoting core strength, stability, and overall body awareness. By breaking down each phase, this exercise not only builds physical resilience but also enhances coordination and proprioception. This section sets the stage for a comprehensive exploration of the Lift, Twist, Stand principles, serving as the foundation for mastery and transformative fitness experiences.

Importance of Lift, Twist, Stand principles

The Lift, Twist, Stand principles form the core foundation of the Turkish Get-Up, each contributing essential elements to its effectiveness. The "Lift" phase establishes a strong base, engaging key muscle groups and initiating the movement. It builds functional strength and reinforces proper lifting mechanics.

The "Twist" phase focuses on core engagement, promoting stability and flexibility. This component enhances rotational strength and challenges the body's coordination, contributing to overall movement proficiency.

The "Stand" phase completes the sequence, emphasizing balance, control, and mobility. Mastering this phase ensures a safe and controlled ascent, reinforcing proper biomechanics and promoting joint health.

Together, these principles create a holistic approach to fitness, targeting various muscle groups and movement patterns. Beyond the Turkish Get-Up, these principles translate into improved functional strength, enhanced body awareness, and injury prevention in everyday activities. Embracing Lift, Twist, Stand principles fosters a well-rounded approach to fitness, unlocking physical potential and contributing to a resilient, adaptable body.

Chapter 1

Fundamentals of Turkish Get-Up

Breakdown of each phase (Lift, Twist, Stand)

Lift Phase:

Initiation: Proper technique for lifting the weight overhead, engaging core muscles.
Shoulder Stability: Focus on stabilizing the shoulder joint during the lift.
Hip Activation: Emphasizing the recruitment of hip muscles for a stable foundation.
Breathing: Coordination of breath with the lifting motion for enhanced control.

Twist Phase:

Core Engagement: Strengthening the core through controlled rotational movements.
Arm Positioning: Maintaining proper arm alignment to support the twist.
Hip Mobility: Developing flexibility and stability in the hips during the twist.
Eye Focus: Importance of visual focus in aiding balance and coordination.
Stand Phase:

Controlled Ascent: Safely transitioning from the ground to a standing position.
Balance and Coordination: Emphasizing stability and awareness throughout the stand.
Foot Positioning: Proper alignment of the feet for optimal balance.
Joint Alignment: Ensuring joints are stacked and aligned during the standing phase.
Understanding the nuances of each phase is crucial for mastering the Turkish Get-Up. This breakdown provides a detailed guide,

focusing on key elements within the Lift, Twist, and Stand components, fostering a comprehensive understanding of the movement and promoting safe and effective execution.

Body mechanics and alignment

Body Mechanics and Alignment in the Turkish Get-Up:

Neutral Spine:

Emphasize maintaining a neutral spine throughout the movement.
Protects the spine and promotes proper alignment of the vertebral column.
Shoulder Packing:

Engage and pack the shoulders down, promoting stability and reducing strain.

Prevents unnecessary tension in the neck and upper traps.
Hip Hinging:

Initiate movements from the hips, promoting hip hinge mechanics.
Facilitates proper weight distribution and activates posterior chain muscles.

Knee Tracking:

Ensure knees track in line with toes during various phases.
Reduces stress on the knee joint and maintains proper lower body alignment.
Engaged Core:

Keep the core engaged throughout, providing stability and protecting the lower back.
Supports balance and control during twists and transitions.
Foot Placement:

Mindful positioning of the foot for stability and weight distribution.
Aids in maintaining balance and proper joint alignment.

Continuous Breath Control:

Coordinate breath with movements, promoting intra-abdominal pressure.
Enhances stability and supports efficient energy transfer.
Understanding and implementing these body mechanics and alignment principles are essential for maximizing the effectiveness of the Turkish Get-Up. Consistent attention to these details ensures a safe, controlled, and biomechanically sound execution, fostering both strength development and injury prevention.

Chapter 2

Lift Phase

Proper technique for initiating the movement

Proper Technique for Initiating the Turkish Get-Up:

Starting Position:

Begin lying on your back with the weight held in one hand, arm fully extended toward the ceiling.
Legs should be bent, and the foot on the same side as the weight should be planted firmly on the ground.

Two-Handed Roll to Press:

Roll onto your side, using both hands to guide the weight as you transition to a seated position.
Maintain a firm grip on the weight throughout this initial movement.

Brace and Lift:

As you transition to a seated position, brace your core and press through the planted foot.
Simultaneously lift the weight overhead, keeping the arm extended and maintaining a neutral wrist.

Establish Half-Kneeling Position:

Move from the seated position to a half-kneeling stance with the foot on the opposite side of the weight forward.

Ensure the knee is directly above the ankle and the back leg is extended comfortably.
Stand-Up:

Push through the front foot, engaging both legs to stand up.
Maintain a stable core and steady gaze throughout the standing phase.
Tips:

Maintain a smooth, controlled pace, avoiding sudden movements.
Keep the weight directly above the shoulder joint during the lift phase.
Focus on maintaining balance and stability as you progress through each step.
Mastering the initiation sets the tone for the entire Turkish Get-Up, ensuring a seamless flow and optimal engagement of muscles. Regular practice with attention to detail will refine this crucial aspect of the movement.

Key muscles involved

Key Muscles Involved in the Turkish Get-Up:

Core Muscles:

Rectus abdominis, obliques, and transverse abdominis are engaged for stability throughout the movement.
Core strength is vital for maintaining a neutral spine and controlling rotational forces.

Shoulder Muscles:

Deltoids, rotator cuff muscles, and trapezius are activated during the lift and stabilization phases.
Shoulder stability is crucial for safely lifting and holding the weight overhead.

Hip Muscles:

Gluteus maximus, medius, and minimus, as well as hip flexors, are actively involved.
Hip strength and mobility play a key role in transitioning between phases and maintaining proper alignment.
Quadriceps and Hamstrings:

Quadriceps assist in standing up, while hamstrings provide stability during the kneeling and standing phases.
Both muscle groups contribute to controlling the movement and supporting the lower body.

Back Muscles:

Erector spinae and latissimus dorsi are engaged for spinal extension and stabilization.
Back muscles provide support and contribute to maintaining an upright posture.

Scapular Stabilizers:

Muscles like the rhomboids and serratus anterior help stabilize the shoulder blades.
Scapular stability is crucial for proper shoulder mechanics during the lift and twist phases.

Adductors:

Muscles along the inner thigh contribute to stability during the transitions and standing phases.
Adductor strength aids in controlling the movement and maintaining balance.
Understanding the key muscles involved in the Turkish Get-Up allows for targeted training and emphasizes the holistic nature of this exercise, promoting overall strength, stability, and functional movement patterns.

Common mistakes and how to avoid them

Common Mistakes in the Turkish Get-Up and How to Avoid Them:

Rushing Through Movements:

Avoidance: Prioritize a controlled pace, focusing on form and alignment at each phase.
Tip: Emphasize quality over quantity during repetitions.
Neglecting Core Engagement:

Avoidance: Maintain constant core activation throughout the entire movement.
Tip: Imagine bracing your core as if preparing for a light punch.
Poor Shoulder Packing:

Avoidance: Ensure shoulders are packed down away from the ears, reducing strain.
Tip: Actively depress the shoulders before initiating the lift.

Unstable Base During Lift:

Avoidance: Anchor the foot on the same side as the weight firmly on the ground.
Tip: Ground the heel and ensure a stable base before lifting.
Incorrect Arm Alignment:

Avoidance: Keep the arm holding the weight directly above the shoulder joint.
Tip: Focus on a vertical line from the wrist to the shoulder during the lift.
Lack of Hip Engagement:

Avoidance: Ensure active hip engagement, especially during transitions.

Tip: Think about pushing through the hips during the lift and maintaining stability in the kneeling positions.

Loss of Balance During Stand:

Avoidance: Control the stand phase by focusing on balance and even weight distribution.

Tip: Fix your gaze on a stable point and engage your core for better stability.

Poor Transitions:

Avoidance: Smoothly transition between phases, avoiding abrupt movements.

Tip: Practice each transition separately before combining them into a fluid sequence.

Addressing these common mistakes fosters a safer and more effective Turkish Get-Up, allowing for optimal engagement of muscles and minimizing the risk of injury. Regular practice with attention to form is key to mastering this intricate movement.

Chapter 3

Twist phase

Detailed Explanation of the Twist Component in the Turkish Get-Up:

Initiation:

The twist component typically begins when transitioning from the seated position to the half-kneeling stance.
As you move, rotate your upper body, initiating the twist through the core.
Core Engagement:

Throughout the twist, maintain strong core engagement.
This involves activating the obliques and transverse abdominis to stabilize the spine.
Arm Positioning:

The arm opposite to the planted foot stays extended overhead.
The free arm supports the twist, helping to guide and balance the movement.

Eye Focus:

Fix your gaze on the extended arm throughout the twist.
Visual focus aids in maintaining balance and coordination during the rotational movement.
Hip Mobility:

The twist involves controlled rotation of the hips.
Maintain awareness of hip positioning, allowing for a smooth and stable transition.

Half-Kneeling Alignment:

As you complete the twist, ensure proper alignment in the half-kneeling position.
The knee on the side of the planted foot should be directly above the ankle.

Controlled Descent:

When returning from the half-kneeling to the seated position, control the descent of the twist.
Use the core muscles to resist gravity and maintain stability.

Smooth Transition to Stand:

The twist component sets the stage for the stand phase.
Ensure a seamless transition, using the rotational force generated during the twist to aid in standing up.
Breath Coordination:

Coordinate your breath with the twist, inhaling or exhaling at key points.
Proper breath control enhances core stability and overall control.

Practice and Progression:

Begin with mastering the twist in isolation before incorporating it into the full Turkish Get-Up.
Gradually increase the weight as your strength and proficiency improve.
Understanding the intricacies of the twist component is crucial for mastering the Turkish Get-Up. Attention to detail and mindful practice contribute to fluidity and efficiency in executing this phase.

Core engagement and stability

Core Engagement and Stability in the Turkish Get-Up:

Bracing Technique:

Initiate core engagement by contracting the muscles around your midsection.
Imagine tightening your abdominal muscles as if preparing for a light punch.

Continuous Activation:

Maintain a consistent level of core activation throughout the entire movement.
This stability is essential for supporting the spine and controlling the various phases.

Transverse Abdominis Focus:

Emphasize contraction of the transverse abdominis, the deep abdominal muscle.
This muscle acts like a natural corset, providing internal support and stability.

Breath Coordination:

Sync your breath with your movements to enhance core stability.
Exhale during exertion phases, such as the lift and stand, for better intra-abdominal pressure.

Oblique Engagement:

The twisting component involves the obliques, so ensure lateral core muscles are actively engaged.
This contributes to rotational stability and control.

Pelvic Floor Activation:

Include the pelvic floor in your core engagement strategy.
Lift and engage the pelvic floor muscles to support the lower abdomen and spine.
Maintaining Neutral Spine:

Focus on preserving a neutral spine, avoiding excessive arching or rounding.
A neutral spine position enhances core stability and reduces the risk of injury.

Integration with Limb Movements:

Coordinate core engagement with movements of the limbs.
For example, actively engage the core when lifting the weight overhead or transitioning between phases.

Progressive Loading:

Gradually increase the load to challenge core stability progressively.
This ensures continued development of strength and endurance in the core muscles.

Mindful Repetition:

During each repetition, consciously assess and maintain core engagement.

Mindful practice reinforces proper muscle activation patterns.

Incorporating these principles into your Turkish Get-Up routine promotes a strong and stable core. Consistent attention to core engagement not only enhances the effectiveness of the exercise but also contributes to improved overall functional fitness and injury prevention.

Progressions for mastering the twist

Progressions for Mastering the Twist in the

Turkish Get-Up:

Isolated Twist Practice:

Begin by practicing the twist component in isolation without the full Turkish Get-Up.

Focus on controlled rotational movements to build familiarity with the twist.

Bodyweight Half-Kneeling Rotation:

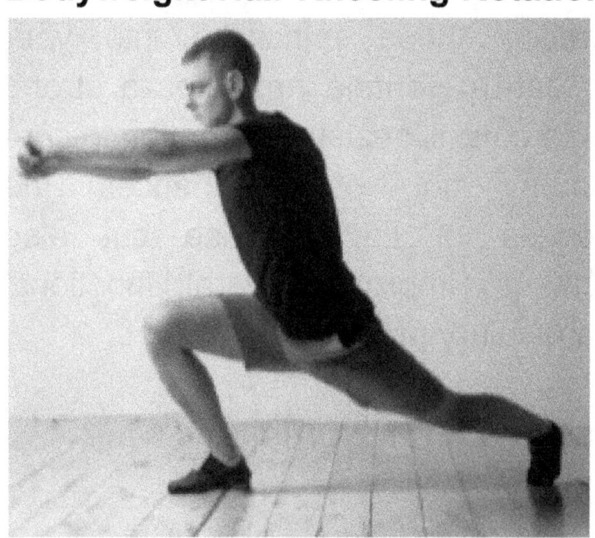

Assume a half-kneeling position without weight.
Rotate the upper body, placing emphasis on core engagement and stability.
Gradually increase the range of motion as comfort and control improve.

Light Weight Half-Kneeling Twist:

Introduce a light weight held with both hands in a goblet position.
Execute the half-kneeling twist with the added challenge of weight.
Ensure smooth transitions between sides.

Single-Arm Overhead Reach:

Lie on your back with the weight overhead and initiate a controlled twist without rising.
Focus on maintaining stability in the rest of the body while emphasizing the rotational aspect.

Half Turkish Get-Up:

Practice the Turkish Get-Up up to the half-kneeling position.
Emphasize the twist phase, ensuring proper alignment and controlled rotation.

Paused Twist:

Pause at various points during the twist to enhance stability and control.
This helps reinforce proper positioning and engagement throughout the movement.
Elevated Arm Position:

Hold the weight with the arm slightly elevated during the twist.
This variation adds complexity to the movement, requiring increased stability.

Dynamic Twist with Momentum:

Incorporate a controlled dynamic twist with a slight momentum.
This progression challenges your ability to manage rotational forces while maintaining stability.

Alternate-Side Turkish Get-Up:

Perform the full Turkish Get-Up but alternate sides with each repetition.

This increases the frequency of twist practice and aids in skill transfer between sides.

Increased Load:

Gradually increase the weight as you become proficient in the twist component.

Ensure that form and stability are maintained with each incremental increase in load.

These progressions allow for a systematic approach to mastering the twist in the Turkish Get-Up, ensuring a gradual build-up of strength, stability, and rotational control. Regular practice and attention to form during each progression contribute to a well-executed and effective twist in the complete movement.

Core engagement and stability

Core Engagement and Stability in the
Turkish Get-Up:

Bracing Technique:

Initiate core engagement by tightening the
abdominal muscles.
Imagine pulling your belly button towards
your spine to activate the deeper core
muscles.

Continuous Activation:

Maintain a consistent level of core activation
throughout the entire movement.
This stability is crucial for supporting the
spine and controlling the various phases.

Transverse Abdominis Focus:

Emphasize the contraction of the transverse
abdominis, a deep-lying core muscle.

This muscle acts like a natural corset, providing internal support and stability.

Breath Coordination:

Sync your breath with your movements to enhance core stability.
Exhale during exertion phases, like the lift and stand, for better intra-abdominal pressure.

Oblique Engagement:

The twisting component involves the obliques, so ensure lateral core muscles are actively engaged.
This contributes to rotational stability and control.

Pelvic Floor Activation:

Include the pelvic floor in your core engagement strategy.

Lift and engage the pelvic floor muscles to support the lower abdomen and spine.

Maintaining Neutral Spine:

Focus on preserving a neutral spine, avoiding excessive arching or rounding.
A neutral spine position enhances core stability and reduces the risk of injury.
Integration with Limb Movements:

Coordinate core engagement with movements of the limbs.
For example, actively engage the core when lifting the weight overhead or transitioning between phases.

Progressive Loading:

Gradually increase the load to challenge core stability progressively.
This ensures continued development of strength and endurance in the core muscles.

Mindful Repetition:

During each repetition, consciously assess and maintain core engagement.
Mindful practice reinforces proper muscle activation patterns.
Incorporating these principles into your Turkish Get-Up routine promotes a strong and stable core. Consistent attention to core engagement not only enhances the effectiveness of the exercise but also contributes to improved overall functional fitness and injury prevention.

Chapter 4

Stand phase

Techniques for safely standing up during the get-up

Techniques for Safely Standing Up During the Turkish Get-Up:

Foot Positioning:

Ensure a stable base by placing the foot on the same side as the weight flat on the ground.
The knee of the opposite leg should be bent, providing a solid foundation for the stand.

Weight Distribution:

Shift your weight onto the planted foot before attempting to stand.

This helps maintain balance and prevents unnecessary strain on the knees.

Engage Glutes and Quadriceps:

Activate the glute muscles and quadriceps of the standing leg.
This not only provides power for the stand but also enhances stability.

Use Arm for Support:

The arm holding the weight should stay extended overhead for support.
This arm serves as a counterbalance, aiding in stability during the stand.

Drive Through Heel:

Focus on pushing through the heel of the planted foot to stand up.

This engages the posterior chain and ensures a controlled ascent.

Maintain Core Engagement:

Keep the core muscles engaged throughout the standing phase.
This enhances stability and helps prevent excessive arching or rounding of the spine.

Controlled Ascent:

Rise gradually, ensuring a smooth and controlled ascent.
Avoid rushing the stand, maintaining awareness of body positioning.

Stable Gaze:

Fix your gaze on a stable point during the stand.
This assists in maintaining balance and coordination throughout the movement.

Avoid Knee Valgus:

Prevent the knee of the standing leg from collapsing inward (knee valgus).
Maintain proper alignment to protect the knee joint.

Full Extension at the Top:

Stand fully upright, extending the hips and knees.
Achieving full extension ensures proper muscle engagement and joint alignment.

Mindful Descent:

When returning to the ground, lower yourself with control.
Reverse the movements, ensuring a gradual descent to the starting position.

Practice with Bodyweight First:

Master the stand with just your body weight before adding external resistance.
This allows for better technique development and reduces the risk of injury.
By incorporating these techniques into your Turkish Get-Up routine, you ensure a safe and effective standing phase, promoting overall movement proficiency and reducing the risk of injury.

Balance and coordination considerations

Balance and Coordination Considerations in the Turkish Get-Up:

Visual Focus:

Maintain a steady gaze on a fixed point throughout the entire movement.
Visual focus enhances stability and aids in coordination.

Slow and Controlled Movements:

Execute each phase of the Turkish Get-Up with deliberate, controlled movements.
Avoid abrupt or jerky motions, which can compromise balance.

Gradual Progression:

Begin with bodyweight or a light weight before advancing to heavier loads.
Gradual progression allows your body to adapt, improving balance and coordination over time.
Mindful Breathing:

Coordinate your breath with each phase, especially during transitions.

Controlled breathing enhances concentration and stability.

Proprioception Exercises:

Include exercises that enhance proprioception, such as single-leg balances. Improved proprioception contributes to better spatial awareness and balance.

Focus on Hip Stability:

Emphasize hip stability during transitions and standing phases.
Strong, stable hips are crucial for maintaining balance throughout the movement.

Practice Unilateral Movements:

Incorporate unilateral exercises to address imbalances between sides.
This helps improve coordination and symmetry in your movement patterns.
Varied Surface Training:

Progress by practicing the Turkish Get-Up on different surfaces.

This challenges your balance and coordination in varied environments.

Incorporate Kettlebell Halo:

Include exercises like the kettlebell halo to enhance shoulder stability.
Improved shoulder stability contributes to overall movement coordination.

Focus on Core Activation:

Engage your core muscles consistently, especially during twists and transitions.

A stable core serves as a foundation for overall balance.

Single-Leg Variations:

Integrate single-leg variations to further challenge balance.
This includes movements like the single-leg deadlift or lunge.

Consistent Practice:

Regularly practice the Turkish Get-Up to build muscle memory and coordination.
Frequent repetition helps refine movement patterns and improves overall proficiency.
By incorporating these considerations into your training, you can enhance your balance and coordination, ensuring a more effective and controlled execution of the Turkish Get-Up.

Variations for different skill levels

Variations for Different Skill Levels in the Turkish Get-Up:

For Beginners:

Bodyweight Turkish Get-Up:

Master the movement without added weight. Focus on proper form and coordination before progressing.
Two-Handed Kettlebell:

Hold a kettlebell with both hands for added stability.
Ideal for those new to the movement and looking to build strength.

Reduced Range of Motion:

Perform a partial Turkish Get-Up, gradually increasing the range of motion.
Suitable for those working on mobility and stability.

Slow Tempo:

Execute each phase of the Turkish Get-Up at a slower pace.
Enhances control, allowing beginners to focus on form.

For Intermediate Level:

Single-Arm Kettlebell:

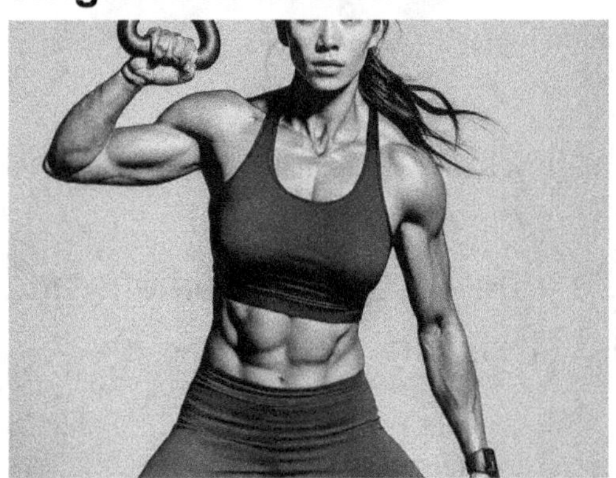

Transition to a single-arm kettlebell for increased challenge.
Requires greater stability and coordination.
Unilateral Load:

Hold a weight in only one hand throughout the entire movement.
Enhances core engagement and balance.
Elevated Arm Position:

Extend the arm holding the weight slightly higher during the movement.
Increases the lever arm, intensifying the challenge.

Paused Repetitions:

Pause briefly at each phase of the Turkish Get-Up.
Builds strength and stability in specific positions.
For Advanced Level:

Bottoms-Up Kettlebell:

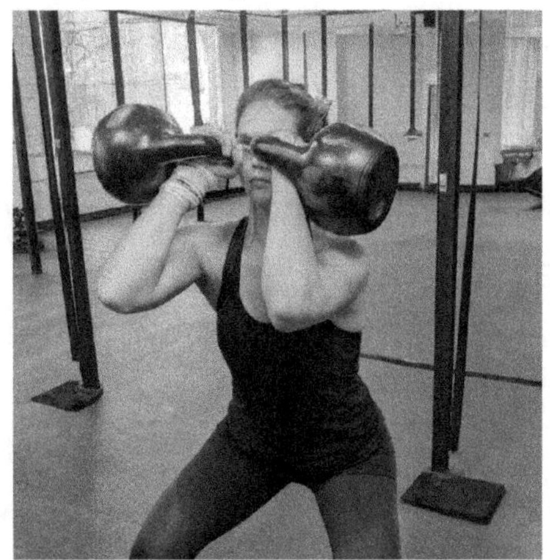

Hold the kettlebell upside down (bottoms-up) for added instability.
Requires exceptional grip strength and shoulder stability.
Heavy Load:

Increase the weight significantly to intensify the challenge.
Suitable for those with a strong foundation in the movement.

Turkish Get-Up to Stand:

Perform the Turkish Get-Up, then transition directly into a standing position.
Adds complexity and requires seamless movement.

Dynamic Turkish Get-Up:

Execute the Turkish Get-Up with a dynamic, explosive lift phase.
Challenges power and coordination.
Tailoring the Turkish Get-Up variations to different skill levels allows for gradual progression and adaptation. Individuals can select the variation that aligns with their current abilities while providing room for continued growth and improvement.

Chapter 5

Integrating Lift, Twist, Stand

Seamless transitions between phases

Tips for Seamless Transitions Between Phases in the Turkish Get-Up:

Fluid Movement:

Aim for a continuous, flowing motion throughout the entire Turkish Get-Up.
Minimize pauses between phases for optimal fluidity.

Maintain Core Engagement:

Keep the core muscles engaged consistently during transitions.
A stable core provides a foundation for smooth movement.

Controlled Breathing:

Coordinate your breath with each transition. Inhale or exhale smoothly, syncing breath with the rhythm of the movement.

Visual Focus:

Maintain a steady gaze on a fixed point. Visual focus enhances coordination and aids in maintaining balance during transitions.

Mindful Awareness:

Stay present and aware of your body's positioning during each phase. Mindful awareness helps prevent unnecessary adjustments between movements.

Practice Slow Transitions:

Initially, practice each transition at a slower pace.
This allows you to refine your technique and build muscle memory.

Weight Distribution:

Distribute your weight evenly during transitions.
Proper weight distribution contributes to stability and controlled movement.

Smooth Handoffs:

Transfer the weight smoothly from one hand to another during phases.
Minimize unnecessary jostling or fumbling with the weight.

Synchronized Limb Movements:

Coordinate movements of the limbs to work harmoniously.
Avoid disjointed or uncoordinated actions for a seamless transition.

Flow Practice:

Incorporate specific sessions focused on enhancing the flow between phases.
Practice the entire Turkish Get-Up as a continuous sequence.

Gradual Progression:

As proficiency improves, gradually increase the speed of transitions.
Ensure that form and control are maintained with each progression.

Visualization:

Mentally rehearse the entire Turkish Get-Up, emphasizing smooth transitions. Visualization can enhance motor control and coordination.
Mastering seamless transitions between phases in the Turkish Get-Up requires a combination of mindful practice, attention to detail, and gradual progression. Consistent effort in refining these elements contributes to a fluid and efficient execution of the movement.

Building fluidity in the Turkish Get-Up

Strategies for Building Fluidity in the Turkish Get-Up:

Consistent Practice:

Regularly incorporate the Turkish Get-Up into your training routine.

Frequent practice reinforces movement patterns and contributes to fluidity.

Mindful Repetition:

Pay close attention to form and technique during each repetition.
Mindful practice helps develop a connection between movements for smoother transitions.

Slow and Controlled Tempo:

Begin with a slower tempo, emphasizing control and precision.
Gradually increase speed as you gain confidence and proficiency.

Connect Phases Seamlessly:

Focus on the seamless flow between each phase of the Turkish Get-Up.
Avoid abrupt movements or pauses, aiming for continuous motion.

Breath Coordination:

Coordinate your breath with each movement, inhaling or exhaling at strategic points.
Proper breath control enhances rhythm and fluidity.

Visualization Techniques:

Mentally rehearse the entire Turkish Get-Up, visualizing smooth transitions.
Visualization can improve motor control and help build a mental map of the movement.
Progressive Loading:

Gradually increase the weight as you become more comfortable with the movement.
This challenges your stability and strength, requiring a more refined and fluid execution.

Flow Workouts:

Design specific workouts focused on continuous flow using the Turkish Get-Up. Perform multiple repetitions in a sequence to enhance overall fluidity.

Smooth Weight Transfers:

Practice transferring the weight smoothly between hands during transitions.
Minimize disruptions to the flow by mastering the handoff technique.
Cueing and Guidance:

Seek feedback from a coach or training partner to identify areas for improvement.
External cues and guidance can enhance your awareness and fluidity.

Address Weak Points:

Identify any specific phases or movements that feel less fluid.

Target those areas with additional attention and practice to improve overall smoothness.

Yoga or Mobility Integration:

Incorporate yoga or mobility exercises to enhance overall body awareness and control.
Improved flexibility and mobility contribute to a more fluid Turkish Get-Up.
Building fluidity in the Turkish Get-Up requires a combination of deliberate practice, attention to detail, and progressive challenges. By incorporating these strategies, you can develop a seamless and graceful execution of this complex movement.

Developing strength and endurance

Strategies for Developing Strength and Endurance in the Turkish Get-Up:

Progressive Load:

Start with a manageable weight and gradually increase it as strength improves. Progressive loading challenges the muscles and promotes strength development.

Higher Repetitions:

Include sessions with higher repetition ranges to enhance muscular endurance. This could involve performing multiple sets of 8-12 repetitions.

Interval Training:

Incorporate interval training with Turkish Get-Ups.
Alternate between periods of higher intensity (heavier weight) and lower intensity

(lighter weight or bodyweight) for endurance benefits.

Complex Training:

Combine Turkish Get-Ups with other exercises in a complex training format.
This approach enhances both strength and endurance by incorporating varied movements.

Tempo Variations:

Experiment with tempo variations, including slower eccentric phases.
Controlled descents during the Turkish Get-Up challenge muscles eccentrically, promoting strength and endurance.

Short Rest Intervals:

Minimize rest intervals between sets to increase the cardiovascular demand.
This approach can enhance overall endurance while still providing a strength stimulus.

Full Range of Motion:

Ensure you're completing the full range of motion during each repetition.
Utilize the entire movement to engage muscles effectively for both strength and endurance.

Unilateral Emphasis:

Focus on unilateral variations, such as single-arm Turkish Get-Ups.
Unilateral work challenges stability and engages muscles for extended periods, promoting endurance.

Circuit Training:

Integrate Turkish Get-Ups into circuit training routines.
Combining the exercise with others maintains an elevated heart rate and builds both strength and endurance.

Increased Training Frequency:

Incorporate Turkish Get-Ups into your training routine more frequently.
Consistent practice improves both strength and endurance over time.

Functional Repetitions:

Perform Turkish Get-Ups with a focus on practical repetitions.
This could involve executing the movement as part of a longer workout to simulate real-world endurance demands.
Periodized Training:

Implement periodization in your training plan.

Periods of higher volume (more repetitions) can target endurance, while lower volume with heavier loads focuses on strength.

Consistent application of these strategies, combined with proper nutrition and recovery, will contribute to the development of both strength and endurance in the Turkish Get-Up. Adjust the variables based on your fitness goals and individual capabilities.

Chapter 6

Troubleshooting common issues

Troubleshooting Common Issues in the Turkish Get-Up:

Issue: Lack of Stability in the Lift Phase

Solution: Ensure a stable base by firmly planting the foot on the same side as the weight. Engage the core and drive through the planted foot during the lift.

Issue: Poor Shoulder Packing

Solution: Actively depress the shoulders away from the ears during the lift. Maintain a strong shoulder position for stability.

Issue: Unstable Base During Stand

Solution: Focus on weight distribution and balance on the standing foot. Engage glutes and quadriceps for a stable ascent.

Issue: Incorrect Arm Alignment

Solution: Keep the arm holding the weight directly above the shoulder joint. Avoid letting the weight drift away from the body.

Issue: Loss of Balance During Twist

Solution: Maintain a stable core and engage the obliques during the twist. Fix your gaze on the extended arm to aid balance.
Issue: Rushing Through Movements

Solution: Prioritize a controlled pace. Slow down and focus on proper form at each phase of the Turkish Get-Up.

Issue: Lack of Core Engagement

Solution: Emphasize constant core activation throughout the entire movement. Brace the core as if preparing for a light punch.

Issue: Excessive Arching or Rounding of the Spine

Solution: Focus on maintaining a neutral spine throughout the Turkish Get-Up. Engage the core to prevent excessive curvature.

Issue: Knee Valgus During Stand

Solution: Ensure proper knee alignment by preventing the knee from collapsing inward. Engage the glutes and maintain a strong, stable stance.

Issue: Uncontrolled Descent

Solution: Lower yourself with control, resisting gravity during the descent. Use the core muscles to maintain stability.

Issue: Inconsistent Breath Control

Solution: Coordinate your breath with each phase. Inhale or exhale at key points, enhancing core stability and overall control.

Issue: Neglecting Progressions

Solution: Gradually progress through variations and challenges. Master each phase before advancing to more complex versions to build a strong foundation.
Regularly assess and address these common issues to refine your Turkish Get-Up technique. Paying attention to details and making corrections will contribute to a safer and more effective execution of the movement.

Adjustments for individual differences

Adjustments for Individual Differences in the Turkish Get-Up:

Mobility Limitations:

Adjustment: Modify the range of motion based on individual flexibility.
Tip: Use props or elevate the hand during the lift phase to accommodate limited shoulder mobility.

Joint Issues or Pain:

Adjustment: Choose a variation that minimizes stress on problematic joints.
Tip: Opt for reduced load or perform partial ranges of motion to avoid exacerbating pain.

Strength Disparities Between Sides:

Adjustment: Focus on unilateral variations to address strength imbalances.
Tip: Perform additional repetitions or sets on the weaker side to promote balance.

Injury History:

Adjustment: Modify the Turkish Get-Up to avoid aggravating previous injuries.
Tip: Consult with a healthcare professional for personalized modifications based on injury history.

Body Size and Structure:

Adjustment: Adapt hand and foot placements based on individual proportions.
Tip: Experiment with positioning to find the most comfortable and effective stance for your body.

Strength Level:

Adjustment: Begin with a weight that aligns with your current strength level.
Tip: Gradually increase the load as strength improves, maintaining a challenging yet manageable progression.

Cardiovascular Endurance:

Adjustment: Adjust the pace and intensity based on individual cardiovascular fitness.
Tip: Shorten rest intervals between sets for a more cardiovascularly demanding workout.

Age-Related Considerations:

Adjustment: Modify the intensity and volume based on age-related factors.
Tip: Focus on controlled movements and prioritize joint health for older individuals.

Skill Level:

Adjustment: Choose a Turkish Get-Up variation that aligns with your current skill level.
Tip: Gradually advance to more complex versions as proficiency improves.

Time Constraints:

Adjustment: Modify the workout duration based on available time.
Tip: Opt for shorter, more intense sessions if time is limited.

Personal Goals:

Adjustment: Tailor the Turkish Get-Up routine to align with individual fitness goals.
Tip: Adjust the number of repetitions, sets, and variations based on whether the emphasis is on strength, endurance, or a combination.

Pre-existing Conditions:

Adjustment: Consider any pre-existing health conditions or concerns.
Tip: Consult with a healthcare professional to ensure that the Turkish Get-Up aligns with your specific health situation.
Customizing the Turkish Get-Up based on individual differences ensures a safe, effective, and personalized training experience. It allows for adjustments that accommodate unique needs, promoting consistency and long-term adherence to the exercise.

Injury prevention tips

Injury Prevention Tips for the Turkish Get-Up:

Proper Warm-Up:

Tip: Begin your workout with a dynamic warm-up to increase blood flow and prepare the muscles and joints for the Turkish Get-Up.

Gradual Progression:

Tip: Progressively increase the weight and complexity of the Turkish Get-Up to allow your body to adapt gradually.

Focus on Technique:

Tip: Prioritize proper form over heavy weights. Ensure each phase is executed with precision to minimize the risk of injury.

Listen to Your Body:

Tip: Pay attention to any discomfort or pain during the exercise. If something doesn't feel right, modify or stop the movement.

Core Engagement:

Tip: Maintain constant core engagement throughout the Turkish Get-Up to provide stability and protect the spine.

Joint Alignment:

Tip: Ensure proper joint alignment during each phase. Avoid excessive twisting or awkward angles that may strain joints.

Warm Down:

Tip: Include a cool-down routine to help relax the muscles and reduce the risk of post-exercise soreness.

Balanced Strength:

Tip: Address muscle imbalances through balanced training. Strengthen opposing muscle groups to maintain joint stability.

Mobility Training:

Tip: Incorporate mobility exercises into your routine to improve joint range of motion, reducing the risk of strains and sprains.

Foot Positioning:

Tip: Ensure stable foot positioning during the Turkish Get-Up. A solid foundation is essential for injury prevention.

Adequate Rest:

Tip: Allow sufficient rest between sets and workouts to prevent overtraining and reduce the risk of fatigue-related injuries.

Hydration and Nutrition:

Tip: Stay hydrated and maintain a balanced diet to support overall health and recovery, reducing the risk of muscle-related injuries.
Consult a Professional:

Chapter 7
Advanced Variations

Progressions beyond the basic Turkish Get-Up

Tip: If you have pre-existing health conditions or concerns, consult with a healthcare professional or fitness expert before incorporating the Turkish Get-Up into your routine.

Variation and Cross-Training:

Tip: Include a variety of exercises and modalities in your training regimen to prevent overuse injuries and promote overall fitness.

Recovery Strategies:

Tip: Incorporate recovery strategies such as foam rolling, stretching, and massage to aid in muscle recovery and prevent tightness.

By integrating these injury prevention tips into your Turkish Get-Up routine, you create a foundation for safe and effective training. Always prioritize your safety and well-being, and seek guidance from fitness professionals if needed.

Training for specific goals

Training for Specific Goals with the Turkish Get-Up:

Strength Development:

Approach: Focus on higher resistance and lower rep ranges.
Tip: Gradually increase the weight, emphasizing proper form to build overall strength.
Muscular Endurance:

Approach: Perform moderate to high repetitions with a manageable weight.
Tip: Use interval training or circuit formats to enhance endurance while maintaining good technique.

Weight Loss and Fat Burning:

Approach: Incorporate the Turkish Get-Up into a high-intensity interval training (HIIT) routine.
Tip: Combine with other full-body exercises for a comprehensive calorie-burning workout.

Core Strength and Stability:

Approach: Emphasize slow and controlled movements, focusing on core engagement.
Tip: Integrate variations that challenge core stability, such as single-arm or bottoms-up kettlebell Turkish Get-Ups.
Improved Mobility:

Approach: Prioritize full range of motion during each phase.

Tip: Include dynamic stretches and mobility exercises in your warm-up and cool-down routine.

Balance and Coordination:

Approach: Incorporate unilateral variations and slow tempo movements.

Tip: Practice Turkish Get-Ups on different surfaces to challenge balance and coordination.

Functional Fitness:

Approach: Mimic real-life movements by incorporating the Turkish Get-Up into a total-body workout.

Tip: Include variations that simulate everyday activities, enhancing functional fitness.

Power and Explosiveness:

Approach: Integrate explosive lifts and dynamic variations.
Tip: Perform Turkish Get-Ups with a faster lift phase, emphasizing power generation.
Sport-Specific Training:

Approach: Customize your Turkish Get-Up routine to complement the demands of your sport.
Tip: Analyze movement patterns in your sport and tailor your training accordingly.
Injury Rehabilitation:

Approach: Consult with a healthcare professional to design a rehabilitation program.
Tip: Use light resistance and controlled movements, gradually increasing intensity as advised by your healthcare provider.
Overall Functional Fitness:

Approach: Include a well-rounded mix of strength, endurance, and mobility work.

Tip: Regularly assess and adjust your training to ensure a balanced and holistic approach to fitness.
Progression and Skill Mastery:

Approach: Systematically progress through variations, focusing on skill refinement.
Tip: Set specific milestones for mastering each phase of the Turkish Get-Up.
Tailor your Turkish Get-Up training to align with your specific goals by adjusting variables like resistance, rep ranges, and movement speed. Periodically reassess your progress and make adjustments to keep your training effective and aligned with your objectives.

Chapter 8

Programming and Training Plans

Structuring workouts incorporating the Turkish Get-Up

1. Warm-Up (5-10 minutes):

Dynamic stretching and joint mobility exercises.
Cardiovascular warm-up with light aerobic activity.

2. Turkish Get-Up Skill Practice (5 minutes):

Focus on refining technique and familiarizing yourself with the movement.
Use a light weight or bodyweight for skill practice.

3. **Main Workout:**

a. Strength Emphasis (Option 1):
- Exercise 1: Turkish Get-Up - 3 sets x 5 reps per side (moderate weight).
- Exercise 2: Goblet Squats - 3 sets x 10 reps.
- Exercise 3: Bent-Over Rows - 3 sets x 8 reps per arm.

b. Endurance Emphasis (Option 2):
- Exercise 1: Turkish Get-Up - 3 sets x 8-10 reps per side (light to moderate weight).
- Exercise 2: Kettlebell Swings - 3 sets x 15-20 reps.
- Exercise 3: Jumping Lunges - 3 sets x 12 reps per leg.

c. Full-Body Functional (Option 3):

- Exercise 1: Turkish Get-Up to Stand - 4 sets x 3 reps per side.
- Exercise 2: Medicine Ball Slams - 4 sets x 15 reps.
- Exercise 3: TRX Rows - 4 sets x 12 reps.

4. Core and Stability Circuit (10 minutes):

Exercise 1: Plank Variations (front plank, side plank) - 3 sets x 30 seconds each.
Exercise 2: Russian Twists - 3 sets x 20 reps.
Exercise 3: Stability Ball Rollouts - 3 sets x 12 reps.

5. Cardiovascular Finisher (5-10 minutes):

High-Intensity Interval Training (HIIT) incorporating bodyweight exercises or cardio equipment.

6. Cool Down and Stretching (5-10 minutes):

Static stretching focusing on major muscle groups used during the workout.
Deep breathing and relaxation.

Notes:

Choose the workout option based on your current fitness level and goals.
Adjust weights and repetitions according to your individual capabilities.
Rest for 60-90 seconds between sets, longer if needed.
Ensure proper form throughout the workout, especially during the Turkish Get-Up.
Listen to your body and modify exercises if necessary.
This structured workout provides a balanced approach, combining strength, endurance, and functional movements. Adjust the intensity and volume based on your fitness level and specific objectives.

Frequency, intensity, and volume considerations

Frequency, intensity, and volume are crucial aspects to consider when incorporating Turkish get-ups (TGUs) into your workout routine.

Frequency:

Beginners may benefit from 1 to 2 sessions per week to allow adequate recovery.
Intermediate and advanced practitioners might aim for 2 to 3 sessions weekly, ensuring ample recovery time between sessions.
Listen to your body; if you experience excessive soreness or fatigue, consider adjusting the frequency.

Intensity:

Start with a weight that allows you to perform the movement with proper form. Technique is paramount in TGUs.
As you progress, gradually increase the weight, focusing on maintaining control throughout the entire movement.
Use a weight that challenges you without sacrificing form. This ensures both safety and effectiveness.
Consider incorporating lighter sessions for skill refinement and heavier sessions for strength development.

Volume:

Beginners might start with 3 to 5 repetitions per side, gradually increasing as they become more comfortable with the movement.

Intermediate individuals can aim for 5 to 8 repetitions per side, adjusting based on individual fitness levels and goals.

Advanced practitioners might incorporate higher volumes, incorporating variations or additional sets to increase the overall workload.

Be mindful of the cumulative volume across your entire workout routine to prevent overtraining.

Progression:

Progression in TGUs can occur through various means – increasing weight, improving form, or incorporating variations.

Gradually introduce changes to keep the routine challenging, such as using a different implement (e.g., kettlebell, dumbbell) or altering the starting position.

Regularly assess your strength and skill level to adjust intensity and volume accordingly.

Recovery:

Adequate rest between sessions is crucial for recovery and preventing overtraining.
Pay attention to your body's signals. If you experience persistent fatigue, soreness, or decreased performance, consider adjusting your training frequency or intensity.
Include mobility work and stretching in your routine to support recovery and reduce the risk of injuries.
Remember, individual responses to frequency, intensity, and volume can vary, so it's essential to listen to your body, progress at a suitable pace, and seek guidance from a fitness professional if needed.

Sample training plans for various levels

Certainly! Here are sample Turkish Get-Up training plans tailored for different levels of fitness:

Beginner:

Frequency: 2 sessions per week

Session Structure:

Warm-up (5-10 minutes of light cardio and dynamic stretching)
Turkish Get-Up Practice:
Start with bodyweight or a very light kettlebell.
Perform 3 sets of 5 reps per side.

Core and Mobility Work:
Planks: 3 sets of 30 seconds.

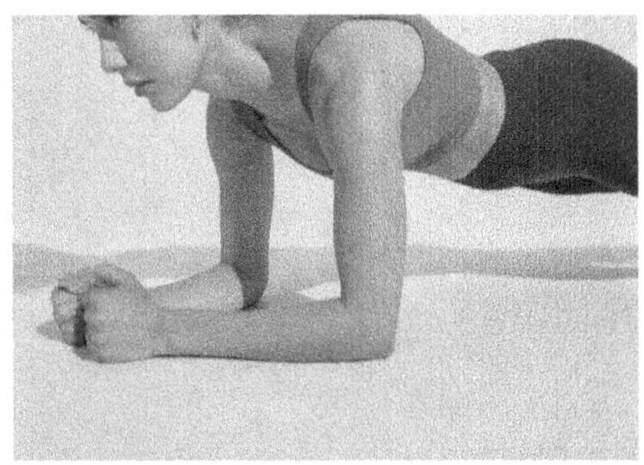

Hip flexor stretches: 2 sets of 60 seconds per side.

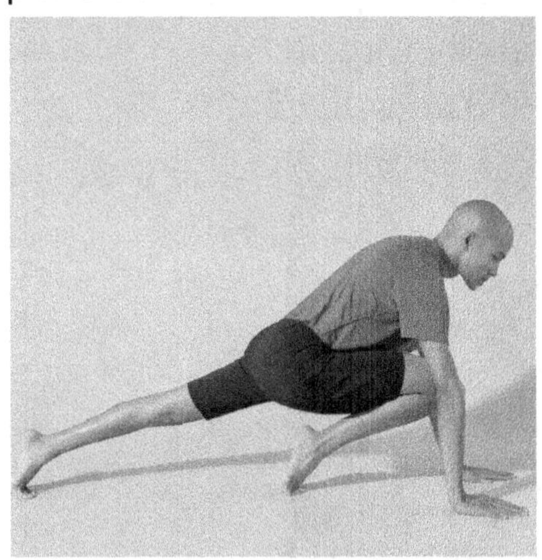

Cool Down (static stretching focusing on shoulders, hips, and core)

Intermediate:

Frequency: 3 sessions per week

Session Structure:

Warm-up (5-10 minutes of light cardio and dynamic stretching)
Turkish Get-Up Practice:
Use a moderate-weight kettlebell.
Perform 4 sets of 6 reps per side.
Strength and Stability Circuit:
Kettlebell swings: 3 sets of 15 reps.

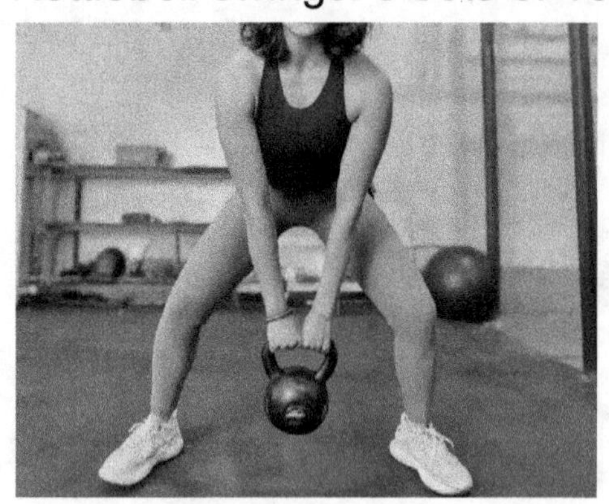

Goblet squats: 3 sets of 12 reps.

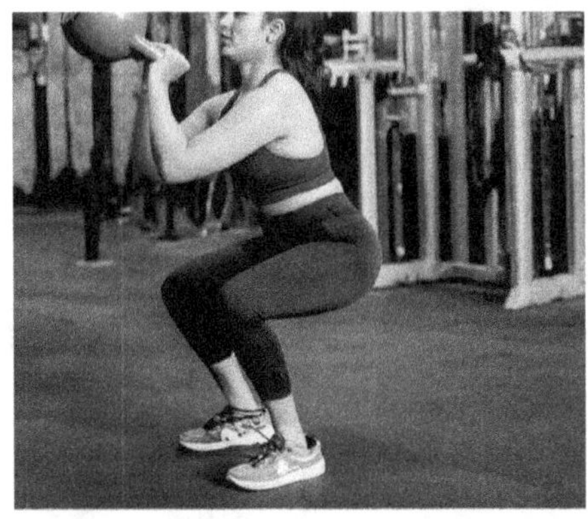

Single-arm rows: 3 sets of 10 reps per arm.
Core and Mobility Work:
Planks variations: 3 sets of 45 seconds.

Spiderman lunges: 2 sets of 10 reps per side.

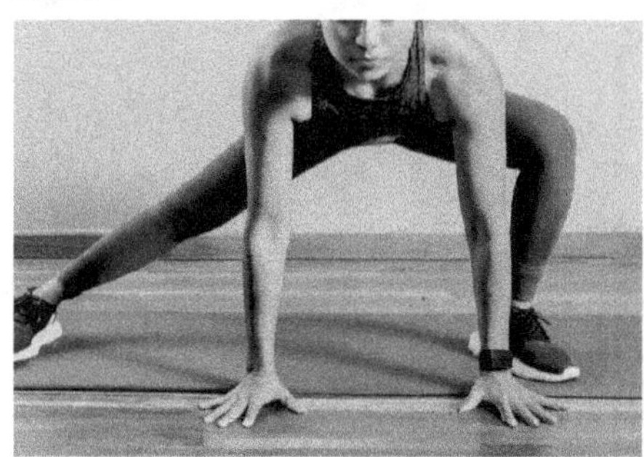

Cool Down (dynamic stretches and foam rolling)
Advanced:

Frequency: 4 sessions per week

Session Structure:

Warm-up (10-15 minutes of light cardio and dynamic stretching)
Turkish Get-Up Practice:
Use a challenging kettlebell.
Perform 5 sets of 8 reps per side.

Complex Strength Circuit:

Turkish Get-Up variations (adding challenges like pauses or slow descent): 3 sets of 5 reps per side.

Overhead squats: 3 sets of 8 reps.

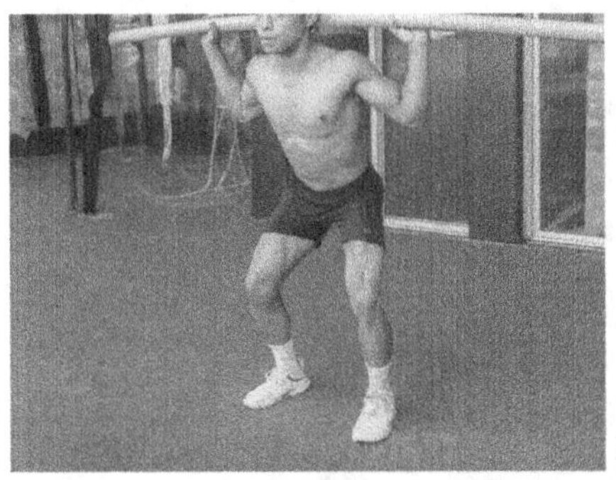

Renegade rows: 3 sets of 10 reps per arm.

Power and Endurance:

Kettlebell snatches: 3 sets of 10 reps per arm.

Farmer's walks: 4 sets of 60 seconds.

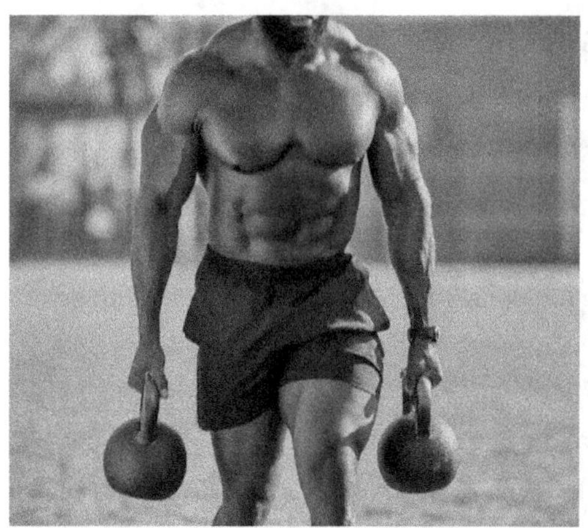

Core and Mobility Work:
Dragon flags: 3 sets of 8 reps.
Dynamic lunges: 2 sets of 12 reps per leg.
Cool Down (yoga-inspired stretches and self-myofascial release)
These plans are just examples, and you should adjust the intensity and volume based on your individual fitness level, recovery capacity, and overall training goals. Always prioritize proper form and listen to your body. Consulting with a fitness

professional can provide personalized guidance.

Chapter 9

Benefits of Mastering the Turkish Get-Up

Physical and mental benefits

Turkish Get-Ups (TGUs) offer a range of physical and mental benefits:

Physical Benefits:

Full-Body Strength: TGUs engage multiple muscle groups, promoting overall strength development. This includes the shoulders, core, legs, and stabilizing muscles.

Functional Movement: The TGU is a complex movement that mimics real-life activities, enhancing functional fitness and improving coordination.

Joint Stability: The controlled movements in TGUs require joint stability, contributing to improved joint health, especially in the shoulders and hips.

Core Strengthening: TGUs place a significant demand on the core muscles, promoting stability and strength in the abdominal and lower back regions.

Improved Posture: The focus on maintaining proper alignment during the movement contributes to better posture and body awareness.

Enhanced Mobility: The TGU involves a variety of movements that encourage flexibility and mobility in the shoulders, hips, and thoracic spine.

Increased Grip Strength: Holding onto the kettlebell during the exercise helps improve grip strength over time.

Cardiovascular Endurance: Performing TGUs with a moderate to heavy load can elevate heart rate, contributing to cardiovascular conditioning.

Mental Benefits:

Focus and Concentration: Executing the TGU requires concentration and mental focus, promoting mindfulness during the workout.

Mind-Body Connection: The intricate movements of the TGU foster a strong connection between the mind and body, enhancing overall body awareness.

Stress Reduction: Engaging in a structured and challenging exercise like the TGU can help reduce stress levels through physical exertion and the focus required.

Confidence Building: Mastering the TGU, especially with progressively heavier weights, can boost self-confidence and a sense of accomplishment.

Patience and Persistence: Learning and refining the TGU may require patience and persistence, teaching valuable lessons in goal-setting and perseverance.

Mental Toughness: Pushing through a set of TGUs, particularly with heavier weights, cultivates mental resilience and toughness.

Variety and Enjoyment: The dynamic nature of TGUs adds variety to a workout routine, potentially increasing enjoyment and adherence to exercise.

Incorporating Turkish Get-Ups into a well-rounded fitness program can contribute to both physical and mental well-being. As with any exercise, it's essential to start at an appropriate level, progress gradually, and prioritize proper form to maximize the benefits while minimizing the risk of injury.

Application to other fitness modalities

The principles and movements involved in Turkish Get-Ups (TGUs) can be applied and integrated into various fitness modalities, enhancing overall functional fitness and performance. Here's how TGUs can complement different exercise approaches:

Strength Training:

TGUs are an excellent compound movement that engages multiple muscle groups simultaneously. They can be integrated into strength training routines as a foundational exercise for full-body strength development.

Kettlebell Training:

TGUs are a staple in kettlebell training. They improve kettlebell skills, grip strength, and dynamic movement control. Combining TGUs with other kettlebell exercises creates a comprehensive and challenging workout.
Functional Fitness:

As a complex, multi-joint movement, TGUs promote functional fitness by mimicking real-world activities. The skills acquired during TGUs, such as stability and coordination, transfer well to daily tasks and activities.

CrossFit:

TGUs can be integrated into CrossFit workouts as a skill-based movement that complements the variety of exercises typically performed in CrossFit training. They contribute to improving overall mobility and strength.

Mobility and Flexibility Training:

TGUs involve a range of movements that contribute to increased flexibility and mobility, especially in the shoulders, hips, and thoracic spine. Integrating TGUs into mobility routines can enhance overall joint health.

High-Intensity Interval Training (HIIT):

Incorporating TGUs into HIIT workouts can add a strength and stability component to the high-intensity sessions. It provides a unique challenge during intervals and contributes to cardiovascular conditioning.

Yoga and Pilates:

The controlled and mindful nature of TGUs aligns well with the principles of yoga and Pilates. Integrating TGUs into these practices can enhance core strength, stability, and body awareness.

Athletic Performance Training:

TGUs are valuable for athletes as they enhance overall body strength, stability, and coordination. They can be incorporated into sports-specific training programs to improve movement patterns and reduce the risk of injuries.

Bodyweight Training:

Even without external resistance, the TGU can be adapted using bodyweight alone, making it suitable for bodyweight training programs. It challenges stability and strength without the need for additional equipment.

Rehabilitation and Injury Prevention:

The controlled and deliberate movements in TGUs make them suitable for rehabilitation programs. They can be used to improve joint stability, correct imbalances, and prevent injuries when incorporated into a well-designed rehabilitation plan.
When applying TGUs to different modalities, it's essential to tailor the intensity, volume, and complexity based on individual fitness levels and goals. Additionally, ensuring proper form and technique remains paramount to reap the full benefits while minimizing the risk of injury.

Frequently asked questions

1. What muscles do Turkish Get-Ups work?

Turkish Get-Ups engage a variety of muscles, including the shoulders, triceps, core, glutes, hamstrings, and stabilizing muscles throughout the body.

2. How often should I do Turkish Get-Ups?

Frequency depends on your fitness level. Beginners can start with 1-2 sessions per week, while intermediate and advanced individuals may aim for 2-4 sessions weekly. Listen to your body and adjust accordingly.

3. Can I do Turkish Get-Ups with bodyweight only?

Yes, you can. Starting with bodyweight helps perfect the movement. As you progress, you can gradually add external resistance like kettlebells or dumbbells.

4. Are Turkish Get-Ups suitable for beginners?

Yes, but it's crucial to start with proper form and a manageable weight. Consider seeking guidance from a fitness professional to ensure correct execution.

5. How heavy should the kettlebell be for Turkish Get-Ups?

Start with a light kettlebell to focus on form. As you become more comfortable, gradually increase the weight. Choose a weight that challenges you without compromising technique.

6. Can Turkish Get-Ups help with weight loss?

Yes, Turkish Get-Ups can contribute to weight loss by increasing calorie expenditure and engaging multiple muscle groups, promoting overall metabolic activity.

7. How long does it take to see results from Turkish Get-Ups?

Results vary, but improvements in strength, stability, and posture can be noticeable within a few weeks with consistent practice. Patience and consistency are key.

8. Are Turkish Get-Ups suitable for older adults?

Yes, TGUs can be adapted for various fitness levels, including older adults. It's recommended to start with lighter weights and prioritize proper form.

9. Can I do Turkish Get-Ups if I have shoulder issues?

Consult with a healthcare professional before attempting if you have shoulder issues. Start with light weights and consider modifying the movement to avoid exacerbating any existing conditions.

10. How can I progress with Turkish Get-Ups?

Progress by increasing weight, perfecting form, and incorporating variations. Gradually challenge yourself to enhance strength, stability, and overall performance.

Conclusion

Recap of key principles

Frequency:

Beginners: 1-2 sessions per week.
Intermediate: 2-3 sessions per week.
Advanced: 3-4 sessions per week.
Adjust based on individual recovery and fitness levels.

Intensity:

Start with a weight that allows proper form.
Progress gradually, increasing weight as strength improves.
Focus on maintaining control throughout the entire movement.

Use different variations for added challenges.

Volume:

Beginners: 3-5 reps per side.
Intermediate: 5-8 reps per side.
Advanced: Higher volumes or variations.
Pay attention to cumulative volume across workouts.

Progression:

Increase weight, improve form, or incorporate variations for progression.
Regularly assess strength and skill levels to adjust intensity and volume.

Recovery:

Allow adequate rest between sessions.
Include mobility work and stretching in your routine.

Listen to your body; adjust frequency or intensity if needed.

Full-Body Strength:

Engages multiple muscle groups, promoting overall strength development.
Functional Movement:

Mimics real-life activities, enhancing functional fitness and coordination.
Joint Stability:

Requires stability, contributing to improved joint health, especially in shoulders and hips.

Core Strengthening:

Emphasizes core muscles, promoting stability and strength in the abdominal and lower back regions.

Improved Posture:

Focus on maintaining proper alignment during the movement contributes to better posture.

Enhanced Mobility:

Involves movements that encourage flexibility and mobility, especially in shoulders, hips, and thoracic spine.

Focus and Concentration:

Requires mental focus, promoting mindfulness during the workout.
Confidence Building:

Mastering TGUs, especially with progressively heavier weights, can boost self-confidence.

Stress Reduction:

Engaging in a structured and challenging exercise like the TGU can help reduce stress levels.

Adaptability:

Suitable for various fitness levels and can be adapted for bodyweight training or with external resistance.
Remember, individual responses may vary, so tailor your TGU practice to your fitness level and goals. Always prioritize proper form and technique for optimal results and safety.

Encouragement and motivation for continued practice

Embarking on the journey of incorporating Turkish Get-Ups into your routine is commendable! As you continue your practice, here's some encouragement and

motivation:

Consistency is Key:

Progress may not happen overnight. Stay consistent with your practice, and you'll gradually see improvements in strength, stability, and overall fitness.
Celebrate Small Wins:

Every successful repetition is a step forward. Celebrate the small victories along the way, whether it's mastering a new weight or completing an extra set.
Embrace the Challenge:

The challenge posed by Turkish Get-Ups is an opportunity for growth. Embrace the difficulty as a chance to push your limits and become stronger both physically and mentally.

Variety Keeps It Exciting:

Explore different variations of TGUs to keep your routine interesting. Whether it's changing the starting position or incorporating pauses, variety can add a new dimension to your practice.

Patience is a Virtue:

Rome wasn't built in a day, and neither is mastery of the Turkish Get-Up. Be patient with your progress, and enjoy the journey of continual improvement.

Listen to Your Body:

Pay attention to how your body responds to each session. If you need an extra day of rest or lighter intensity, listen to your body's cues for optimal recovery.
Set Realistic Goals:

Establish achievable short-term and long-term goals. Whether it's increasing the weight or perfecting your form, setting realistic goals keeps you motivated and focused.

Visualize Success:

Envision yourself successfully completing a challenging TGU. Visualization can be a powerful tool to enhance performance and boost confidence.
Community Support:

Share your journey with others, whether it's friends, family, or fellow fitness enthusiasts.

A supportive community can provide motivation and encouragement.
Feel the Progress:

Take note of how your body feels after each session. Increased strength, improved mobility, and enhanced overall well-being are all signs of progress.
You Are Stronger Than You Think:

Your body is capable of incredible feats. Trust in your strength and resilience. With dedication, you'll surprise yourself with what you can achieve.
Remember, your commitment to Turkish Get-Ups is an investment in your health and fitness. Keep pushing yourself, stay positive, and enjoy the journey of continual growth and self-improvement. You've got this!

Request for Review

Dear Reader,

I hope you've found "Lift, Twist, Stand: Mastering the Turkish Get-Up" to be a valuable resource on your journey to mastering this dynamic exercise. Your feedback is immensely important to us, and we would love to hear about your experience with the book.

If you've enjoyed the content, gained insights, or found the information helpful, kindly consider leaving a review. Your thoughts not only contribute to the growth of this guide but also help fellow readers make informed decisions.

Your feedback is highly valued, and we appreciate your time and consideration.

Warm regards,

Helen Talbott